QUICK & EASY
KETO
MEAL PREP

With over 70 Healthy Recipes and Great Meal Plan for Weight Loss to make the start of your journey easier

- VOLUME 1 -

presented by

OLVIDO MENA

TABLE OF CONTENTS

25. Filipino Nilaga Soup
26. Pork Tenderloin with Southern Cabbage
27. Indian-Style Fried Pork

BEEF

28. Italian-Style Spicy Meatballs
29. Rich Double-Cheese Meatloaf
30. Meat and Goat Cheese Stuffed Mushrooms
31. Shredded Beef with Herbs
32. Chinese Ground Beef Skillet
33. Easy Steak Salad
34. Saucy Skirt Steak with Broccoli
35. Classic Beef Stroganoff

FISH & SEAFOOD

36. Catfish and Cauliflower Casserole
37. Swedish Herring Salad
38. Hearty Fisherman's Stew
39. Fish and Vegetable Medley
40. Salmon Curry with a Twist
41. Tuna, Avocado and Ham Wraps
42. Alaskan Cod with Mustard Cream Sauce
43. Smoked Haddock Fish Burgers

EGGS & DAIRY

44. Paprika Omelet with Goat Cheese
45. Dilly Boiled Eggs with Avocado
46. Greek-Style Frittata with Herbs
47. Mangalorean Egg Curry
48. Egg, Bacon and Kale Muffins
49. Cheesy Brussels Sprouts
50. Cauliflower, Cheese and Egg Fat Bombs
51. Double Cheese and Sausage Balls

VEGETARIAN

52. Mexican Inspired Stuffed Peppers
53. Frittata with Asparagus and Halloumi
54. Baked Eggs and Cheese in Avocado
55. Two-Cheese Zucchini Gratin
56. Italian Zuppa di Pomodoro
57. Two-Cheese and Kale Bake
58. Grandma's Zucchini and Spinach Chowder
59. Crêpes with Peanut Butter and Coconut

SNACKS & APPETIZERS
60. Lettuce Wraps with Ham and Cheese
61. Ranch and Blue Cheese Dip
62. Ranch Chicken Wings
63. Colby Cheese-Stuffed Meatballs
64. Cheese and Artichoke Dip
65. Italian Cheese Crisps
66. Deviled Eggs with Mustard and Chives
67. Mini Stuffed Peppers

DESSERTS
68. Almond Butter and Chocolate Cookies
69. Basic Orange Cheesecake
70. Peanut Butter and Chocolate Treat
71. Coconut Cranberry Bars
72. Peanut and Butter Cubes
73. Easiest Brownies Ever
74. No Bake Party Cake
75. Vanilla Mug Cake

INTRODUCTION

I have struggled with my weight almost my whole life, since my teenage years. I've been on a diet since I was 14. I was always hungry; I didn't have a good night's sleep and energy for my daily tasks and activities. Shortly after that, I got stuck in a cycle of "yo-yo dieting" or weight gain followed by weight loss. I spent many years feeling out of control with my eating. I felt that I was disconnected from my own body and I didn't listen to it but I cannot help myself. As a teenager of 16, I struggled with depression. I felt devastated; my friends could not understand how this straight-A student and beautiful girl could have any mental problems. In addition, my parents did not understand what I was going through; they thought I went through a phase like other teens with fluctuating emotions. Later, when I was in college, my struggles continued. I was dieting, sometimes successfully sometimes not. It is like a hamster on its wheel!

When I graduated college, I had everything I thought I wanted. Nevertheless, I wasn't happy. I had an almost phobic fear of food, especially greasy food, nuts, and fatty cheese. This belief about fats is based on a common fact that we have heard so many times so we just assume it is true. It is like many other ideas that fall into the category of "myths" that are totally wrong! Ironically, natural food, including natural fats, is good for the human body. In theory, if you want to lose weight, you should burn more calories than you eat; you should also pay attention to regular physical activities, take the stairs instead of elevators, walk an extra 30 minutes a day, blah, blah, blah… Easier said than done. In practice, we should analyze many factors to understand that there are often more than one cause of weight gain. Psychological factors, genetic predisposition, food addiction, high insulin levels, hormone imbalance, and neurologic problems all may play a part.

When I look back on my life, I see low self-esteem and misery. I also thought that cooking at home is time-consuming so I regularly ordered food delivery. I decided to stop torturing myself and break the starve-binge cycle. I decided to be happy! "Everything in your life is a reflection of a choice you have made. If you want a different result, make a different choice," said Anonymous. So, I asked myself, "What make you feel persistently hungry, despite eating enough food and three meals a day? What are you doing to your body!? What should you do if you want to feel and look your best?" These questions were complicated for me, but deep in my heart, I knew that the answers were simple. Luckily, I found the answers and heal my relationship with food.

Three years ago, I had discovered a low-carb dietary regimen. It is a low carbohydrate, moderate protein, and high fat based diet. Basically, I can eat meat, poultry, eggs and dairy on a keto diet and avoid rice, grains and legumes. I was skeptical at first, it sounds too good to be true! Fortunately, I was proven wrong, this nutrition plan is better than I've ever expected. My goal with this recipe collection is to show you an easy but effective way to kickstart a ketogenic diet. Also, I wanted to use my experience and knowledge to encourage you on your keto adventure with all ins and outs. After years of struggle, I feel optimistic and inspired to pay it forward and help others to find their path to a happy life. If you feel overwhelmed or intimidated, whatever you are going through, I am here to tell you that everything is possible; so, never give up. If I can do it, you can too!

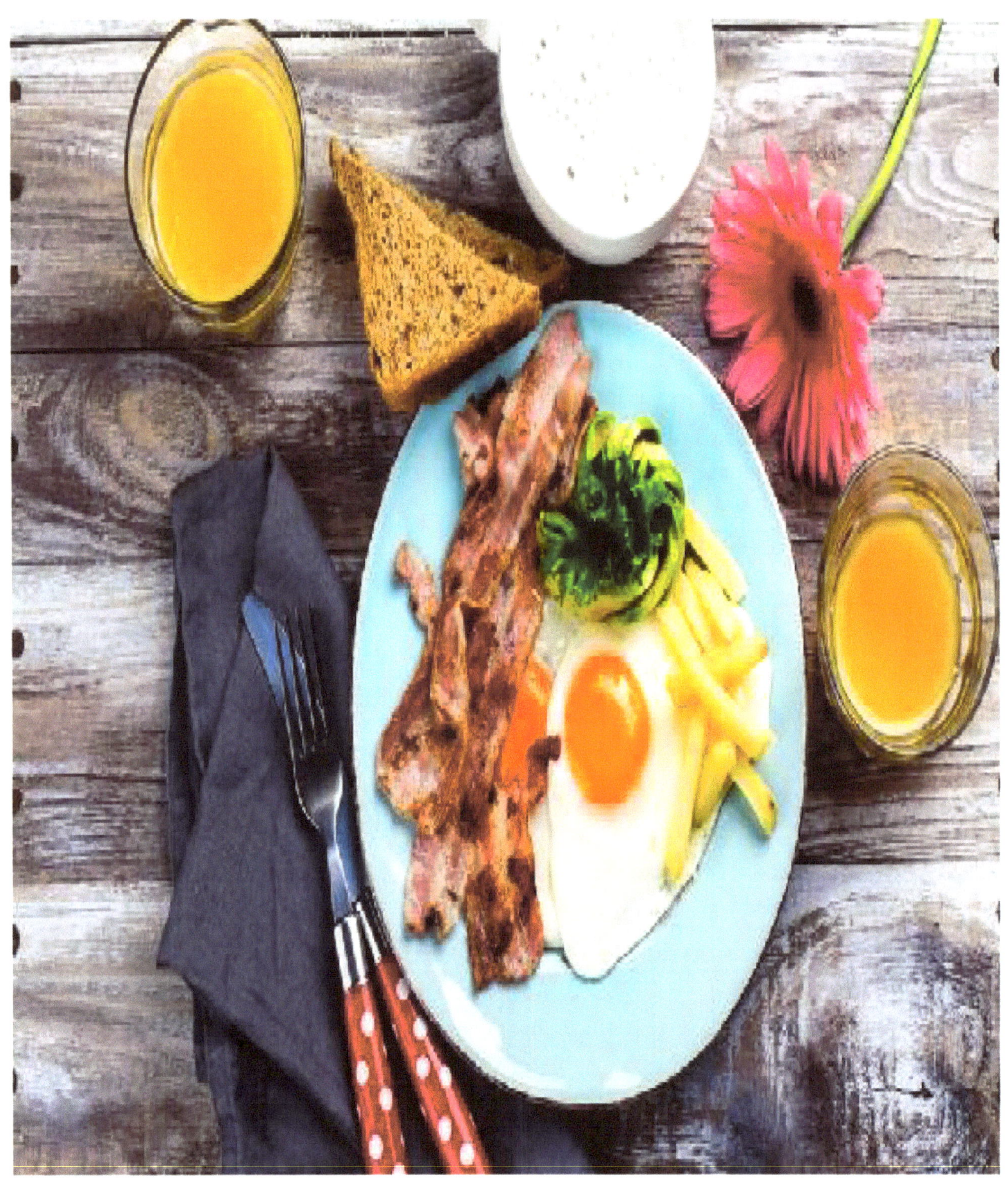

What is the Keto Diet?

According to Wikipedia, "A ketogenic diet is a diet that derives most of its calories from fat and only a small number of calories from carbohydrates. The diet forces the body to burn fats rather than carbohydrates for energy. Normally, the carbohydrates you eat are turned into glucose in the body, which is used for energy around the body and in the brain. But, if you don't eat enough carbohydrates, your body has a back-up system of burning fat instead. The liver can use stored fat and the fat you eat for energy. Stored fat is broken into two parts, fatty acids, and ketone bodies. Ketone bodies power the brain instead of glucose. This state of having a lot of ketone bodies in your blood is called *Ketosis*."

When I discovered a keto lifestyle, something about it really inspired me to do detailed research. I read a lot of articles and studies, seeing real people getting real and great results; then, I put theory into practice and Voilà! I did it! And I did it well! A month after starting this amazing lifestyle, my life completely changed.

I started following a ketogenic diet with a daily calorie breakdown of 5% carbs, 20% protein, and 75% fats. I also tried to stay within my calorie needs. It is not difficult since a common symptom of this diet is the feeling of fullness. The appetite suppression may be linked to a higher intake of fat and protein. My ultimate goal was to boost the body's metabolism to speed up my weight loss. Besides being in ketosis, I tried to make some changes to help rev up my metabolism. Some of these changes include eating a good breakfast, doing simple exercises to build muscles, eating protein with every meal, drinking green tea, and adding hot peppers to my meals. "Do not skip meals" is one of the best tips I've ever heard since skipping meals, especially breakfast, can cause the metabolism to slow down.

Once I reached my ideal weight, I tried to rotate very low carbohydrate days with higher carbohydrate days so I can say that simple plan works for me. Alternatively, you can keep on with your keto lifestyle, but you can eat a little more food for weight maintenance. You can add a little more protein but keep carbs low. You can add more carbs only before and after workouts. It is advisable to go slowly, and raise your daily carb limit by 10 to 20 grams for a week or two, and stick with Paleo foods. In this phase, you can eat carbs that are nutrient-dense and fiber-rich such as carrots, peppers, potatoes, turnips, pears, bananas, oranges, and strawberries. Another great way to maintain your goal weight is to combine intermittent fasting with muscle-gaining keto. The key is just to find that perfect amount of food for your body, age, and activity level. Most people, including me, do not have to be in ketosis to stay at a healthy weight, as long as they stick with a low-carb diet such as Paleo, LCHF or low-carb Mediterranean diet. Almost four years into keto, I am maintaining my ideal weight, feeling freedom from food like the one I have never had before. Pro Tip:

Choose nutrient-packed foods that can satiate you easier, and automatically, you will eat less.

What to Eat on a Ketogenic Diet?

I created a detailed keto-friendly food list so you can keep it in your shopping bag.

<u>Vegetables</u>: Lettuce (all types), greens (spinach, Swiss chard, collard, mustard greens, kale, and turnip); mushrooms, onion, garlic, asparagus, arugula, avocado, celery, squash, kohlrabi, bok choy, radishes, broccoli tomatoes, cauliflower, zucchini, eggplant. In moderation: artichokes, Brussels sprouts, broccolini, cauliflower, cucumbers, green beans, cabbage, okra, snap peas, snow peas, and fennel.

<u>Fruits</u>: Blackberries, cranberries, raspberries, lemon, lime, coconut, and tomatoes.

<u>Meat & Poultry</u>: Beef, pork, game, lamb, and veal, chicken, turkey and duck.

<u>Ground meat</u>: Pork, beef, turkey, and mixed ground meat.

<u>Lunch & Deli Meats</u>: Bacon, pancetta, pepperoni, salami, soppressata, chorizo, ham, pastrami, prosciutto, and speck. In moderation: bologna and mortadella.

<u>Seafood</u>: Fatty fish, white fish, lobster, crab, shrimp, scallops, mussels, squid, oysters, and octopus.

<u>Dairy</u>: Cream cheese, blue cheese, mozzarella, brie, Colby cheese, goat, provolone, Gouda, Muenster, camembert, and Swiss cheese; heavy cream, double cream, half-and-half; butter and ghee; eggs. In moderation: whole milk, cheddar cheese, feta, Pepper Jack cheese, full-fat Greek yogurt, crème fraîche, mascarpone, cottage cheese, sour cream, and ricotta.

<u>Nuts & Seeds</u>: peanuts, almonds, walnuts, Brazil nuts, pecans, hazelnuts, macadamia nuts, pine nuts, chia seeds, hemp seeds, pumpkin seeds, and sunflower seeds.

<u>Fats & Oils</u>: Coconut oil, avocado oil, olive oil, flaxseed oil, cocoa butter, and nut oil; lard, duck fat, schmaltz, and tallow.

<u>Keto-friendly drink options</u>: Coffee, tea, diet soda, seltzer, sparkling water, keto smoothies, zero carb energy drinks.

Other keto-friendly foods include: <u>Herbs and spices</u> (fresh or dried); bouillon cubes and granules.

<u>Sauces & Condiments</u>: Mayonnaise, mustard, tomato sauce, vinegar, and hot sauce (make sure to check the nutrition facts label).

<u>Canned food</u>: tuna anchovies, crab, salmon, sardines, tomato, sauerkraut, pickles, and olives (make sure to check the nutrition facts label).

<u>Baking ingredients</u>: almond flour, coconut flour, baking powder, baking soda, cocoa, vanilla extract, dark chocolate, glucomannan powder.

<u>Nut & Seed Butters</u>: peanut butter, almond butter, hazelnut butter, macadamia nut butter, coconut butter, pecan butter, sunflower seed butter, walnut butter, and tahini.

<u>Vegetarian</u>: Tempeh, tofu, full-fat coconut milk, jackfruit, nutritional yeast, Shirataki noodles, Nori sheets, roasted seaweed, Kelp noodles, Kelp flakes.

<u>Keto-Friendly Alcohol</u>: Whiskey, brandy, dry martini, vodka, and tequila.

<u>Seaweed</u>: Wakame, chlorella, nori, dulse, spirulina, and kelp.

<u>Keto sweeteners</u>: Stevia drops, Erythritol, and Monkfruit are zero carb sweeteners; Splenda (sucralose-based sweetener) has 0.5g of carbs per packet (1 g); Erythritol has 4 grams of carbs per teaspoon (4 grams); Xylitol has 4 grams of carbs per teaspoon (4 grams); **Foods to Avoid on a Ketogenic Diet**

<u>Grains & grain-like seeds</u>: Rice, wheat, quinoa, oats, amaranth, barley, buckwheat, corn, millet <u>Flours</u>: Wheat flour, cornmeal, arrowroot, cornstarch, cassava, dal, and fava beans.

<u>Starches</u>: Starchy vegetables, soy, lentils, sago, tapioca, plantain, banana, and mesquite.

<u>Sugars</u>: All types of sugar and syrup (rice syrup, malt syrup, sorghum syrup, corn syrup, carob syrup, and high maltose corn syrup), barley malt, cane juice crystals, cane juice, treacle, malt, rapadura, muscovado, panocha, scant, agave nectar, molasses, honey, and maple syrup.

<u>Processed vegetable oils & trans fats</u>: Diglycerides, shortening, vegetable shortening, margarine, interesterified oils, corn oil, cottonseed oil, grapeseed oil, safflower oil, and soybean oil.

<u>Milk & reduced-fat dairy products</u>: evaporated skim milk, low-fat yogurts, fat-free butter substitutes, and reduced fat cheese.

<u>Factory-farmed fish and eggs, processed meat</u>

<u>Fruits (other than berries) & dried fruits</u>

<u>Sugary drinks:</u> soda and energy drinks.

Ketogenic Kitchen Makeover

To make your keto grocery shopping easier, here is the list of pantry essentials on a keto diet. It will help you to save money by not buying unnecessary items.

- LOW-CARB FLOURS – Almond flour (1/4 cup or 28 grams of almond flour has around 160 calories and 6 grams of total carbs); Coconut flour (2 tablespoons or 18 grams of coconut flour has around 45 calories and 11 grams of total carbs); Flax meal (2 tablespoons or 14 grams of flax meal has nearly 70 calories and 5 grams of total carbs); Sunflower seed meal and Pumpkin seed meal.

- SWEETENER – Stevia, Xylitol, Erythritol.

- NUTS & SEEDS

- CREAM CHEESE

- COCONUT MILK & COCONUT CREAM

- COCONUT OIL, AVOCADO OIL & OLIVE OIL

- MEAT, POULTRY & SEAFOOD

- NUT BUTTERS

- KETO VEGETABLES & FROZEN VEGETABLES

- CONDIMENTS – Mustard, mayonnaise, Sriracha, hot sauce, and vinegar.

- CACAO POWDER, CACAO NIBS & SUGAR-FREE DARK CHOCOLATE

- PSYLLIUM HUSKS

- HERBS & SPICES – pink salt, sage, thyme, rosemary, black pepper, oregano, basil, ginger, turmeric, and cinnamon.

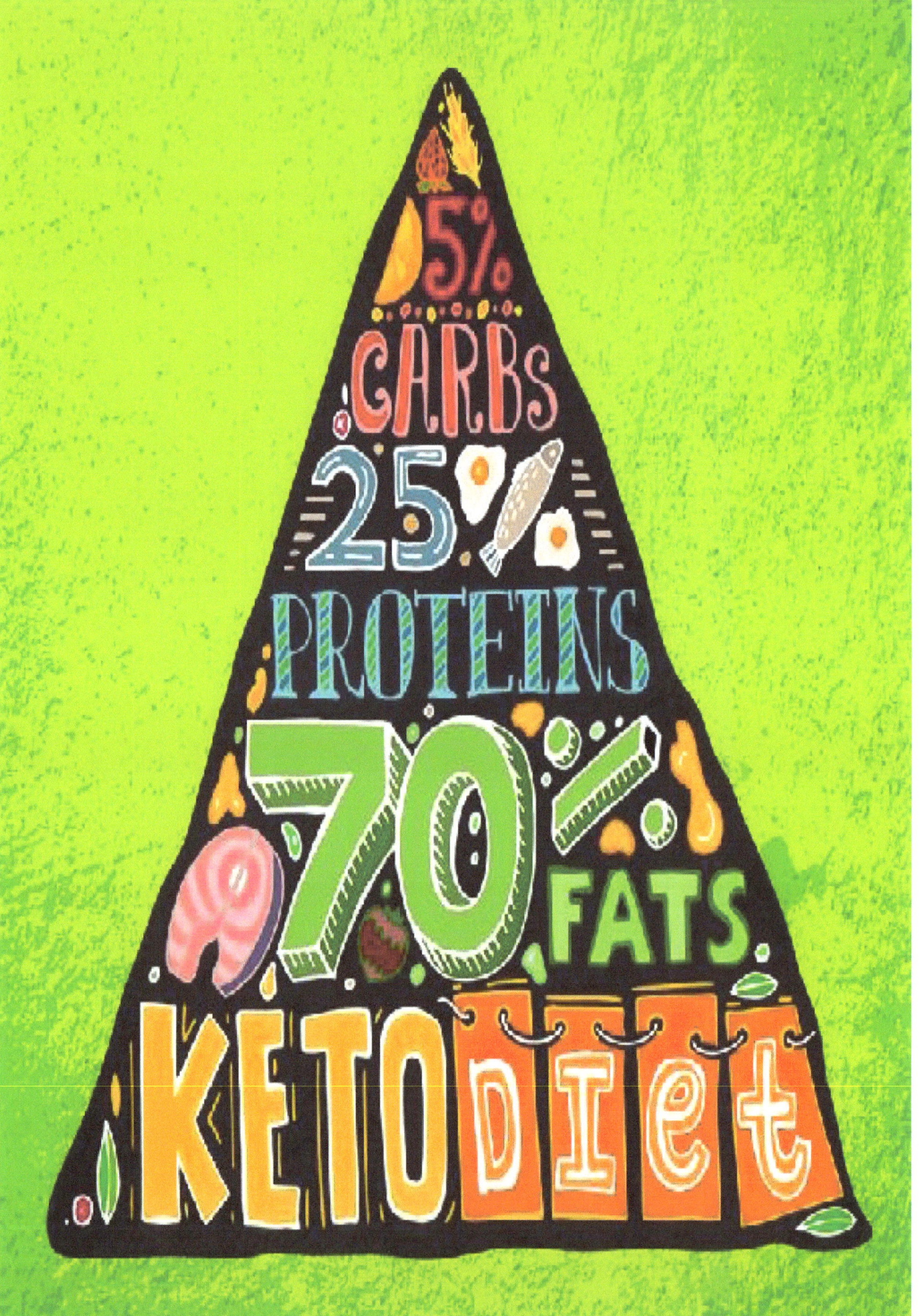

5%
CARBS
25%
PROTEINS
70%
FATS
KETO DIET

Macronutrient Balance

Macronutrients ("macros") include protein, fat, and carbs. Macronutrients provide energy in the form of calories. For instance, fat provides 9 calories per gram; then, there are 4 calories per gram of protein; as for carbohydrates, there are 4 calories per gram. Luckily, you can calculate your keto macros in a couple of minutes by using the Keto Calculator online. It can help you find the exact amount of macronutrients you need to reach your goal, whether you want to lose or maintain your weight. There are calculators for a classic ketogenic diet (75% fat, 20% protein, 5% carbohydrate) and other variations of keto diets so you can input specific amounts of macros according to your preference.

FATS (LIPIDS) are an essential part of a ketogenic diet. The type of fats you eat on a keto diet is essential because some fats are better for weight loss and healthier than others. It took me long to understand that I need to eat fat to burn fat. If you avoid fat and eat large amounts of lean protein foods such as skinless chicken and fish, the excess protein will be converted into glucose. It can raise your insulin levels, too. Low-fat products may seem like a good option for weight loss because fats have been given a bad reputation in the past. However, reduced-fat peanut butter, fat-free salad dressings or low-fat yogurt often contain a lot of unhealthy ingredients, processed oil, and sugar. The trick here is to eat more fat. For example, I'd like to add butter to my breakfast, it fills me up and helps me eat less at lunch. Keep in mind that the human body needs all types of fats including unsaturated fats and saturated fats. There are two main types of unsaturated fats: 1) polyunsaturated fats (include omega-3 fats and omega-6 fats), and 2) monounsaturated fats.

Sources of monounsaturated fatty acids include olive oil, peanut oil, canola oil, sesame oil, and cashews. Foods with a higher amount of polyunsaturated fat include nuts, seeds, soybean oil, and fatty fish. Foods with higher amounts of saturated fats include fatty beef, butter, cheese, pork, poultry with skin, cream, and lard. There is one more category called "Trans fats" that are unsaturated fats that have been processed. You should eat less saturated and trans-fats in order to lower the risk of heart disease, high blood cholesterol, and obesity. To illustrate, junk food and packaged foods contain saturated fat in a larger amount. Therefore, you should avoid snack foods (such as fatty potato chips), fried foods, high fat takeaway foods (including pizza, pasta, hamburgers), high-fat cakes, biscuits, and muffins, pastries (such as pies and croissants). Check the labels and opt for the products that are higher in poly and monounsaturated fats and lower in saturated and trans-fats. Remember, it is important to eat fats in small amounts as a part of a balanced ketogenic diet.

PROTEIN also plays a unique role in the human body. It consists of smaller units called amino acids; you need essential amino acids for your body to function properly. The most important functions of proteins include the creation of hormones, maintaining a healthy weight, promoting longevity, muscle growth and repair. Protein is crucial for a skin, bone, and brain health, too. Animal protein sources on a keto diet include seafood, meat, poultry, cheese, and eggs. Plant protein sources include most nuts and seeds.

There are different views on protein intake on a keto diet. Some ketogenic researchers suggest high protein intake (1 gram of protein per 1 pound). Some experts advocates low protein intake for people who follow a keto diet or 1.0 grams of protein per kilogram of lean mass (2.2 pounds). They believe excess protein can turn into sugar in your body and prevent ketosis. There is the third group of experts that recommends 1.5-1.75 grams of protein per 2.2 pounds. Most people agree that we should follow this formula to enter and stay in ketosis – 5% carbs, 20% protein, and 75% fats.

CARBOHYDRATES are macronutrients that the human body converts to glucose; in fact, glucose is the body's principal fuel source. Your organs such as kidneys, brain, and heart all need carbs to function properly. Furthermore, fats can't be properly metabolized without carbs in the form of fiber that are needed for digestion. Besides being a fuel, glucose can be stored as glycogen in our liver or muscles. Put simply, overconsumption of carbs increases the creation of more fat storage.

The human body also requires micronutrients, including vitamins and minerals. Bear in mind that the majority of micronutrients and important phytonutrients come from vegetables; it means that you should eat a large portion of keto veggies with every meal. When you know your macros, you can easily plan your day on a ketogenic diet.

6 Critical Ketogenic Diet Tips

Eat a solid keto breakfast to lose weight.

You should make time to start your day right. Heaving a good breakfast with protein and healthy fats, such as an omelet or egg muffins, will control your eating throughout the day. Eating a healthy low-carb breakfast can significantly restore the glucose levels in your body just like your car needs fuel to run. You should focus on having protein-rich foods such as milk, nuts, seeds, and eggs. Skipping breakfast affects mood and cognitive function. In addition, it may lead to hypertension, high cholesterol, and high blood pressure. Researches have proven that people who skip breakfast have high levels of fatigue throughout the day.

If you think you have no time for breakfast, this recipe collection may help you to overcome that problem. This collection offers easy breakfast ideas such as egg muffins, keto fat bombs, low-carb pancakes, and so forth. You can also turn dinner leftovers into a go-to breakfast. A casserole with eggs and bacon that is topped with sharp cheese makes a fantastic leisure dinner as well as a grab-and-go breakfast. Make-ahead breakfast is good idea for those short on time, too. For instance, you can make lettuce wraps, chicken salad or cheese crisps and store them in airtight containers up to 3 days. You can make a cheese and vegetable gratin in Sunday morning; it can be reheated quickly or enjoyed cold straight from the refrigerator. With our keto recipes, you can easily make meal prep a habit! Remember, your body needs to refuel first thing in the morning. Therefore, take your breakfast within an hour of waking up. Breakfast is an all-important key to a successful keto diet and to better health.

Learn to use the nutrition facts label.

First things first, keep carbs low. It will help you to make better food choices that contribute to your diet. Then, check for hidden sugars, which is "enemy number one" on a keto diet. Most processed foods contain hidden sugar since it enhances flavor and helps preserve foods. Common sweeteners include raw sugar, brown sugar, sucrose, sugar syrup, high-fructose corn syrup, invert sugar, cane sugar, corn syrup, Turbinado, corn sweetener, dextrose, fructose, fruit juice concentrates, maltose, glucose, lactose, malt syrup, and Sorghum syrup. They don't contribute any health benefits to your meals.

You should also avoid the following ingredients: caramel, cane juice, cane juice solids, dextrin, dextran, barley malt, beet sugar, buttered syrup, carob syrup, date sugar, diatase, diatastic malt, golden syrup, Refiner's syrup, and ethyl maltol. Statistics have shown that the average American consumes at least 64 pounds of sugar per year or 22 teaspoons of added sugars a day. When it comes to healthy keto sweeteners, you should opt for a sweetener that is made of natural ingredients and does not contain chemicals. In addition, you should choose a sweetener that has nutritional value but you'll still be within your daily carb limit. Stevia and monk fruit are natural sweeteners that provide health benefits. Stevia is three hundred times sweeter than sugar and has no impact on blood sugar levels. When purchasing stevia, look for a pure, organic product. Monk fruit is a zero-calorie sweetener; studies have proven that monk fruit has significant anti-inflammatory and antioxidant properties. It is useful in reducing inflammation and regulating insulin tolerance.

Learn how to build muscle on a keto diet.

Building lean mass is crucial for a successful ketogenic diet because you will burn off your body's fat storages more efficiently. There are four types of exercises I did for boosting muscle size: Deadlifts, overhead press, squats, and bench press.

It's important to refuel your body with nutrient-dense keto food for optimal athletic performance. In addition, pay close attention to your electrolyte consumption. For example, low-carb, potassium-rich foods include mushrooms, spinach, broccoli, and salmon. Low-carb, magnesium-rich foods include almonds, avocados, and dark chocolate. The body also loses sodium, chloride, and calcium during exercise.

Calculate net carbs.

I know it can be confusing to figure out how much carbs to incorporate into your daily meal plan. Learning how to calculate net carbs is essential for success on a keto diet. In fact, net carbs are the carbohydrates that our body can digest and uses for energy. Stick to the formula: Total Carbohydrate - Dietary Fiber - Sugar Alcohol = Net Carbs. Dietary fiber and sugar alcohol (most of them) are non-digestible carbs. Your liver does not use non-digestible carbs to convert them into glucose. Therefore, net carbs only count starches and sugars.

In other words, you don't need to include sugar alcohols (xylitol, mannitol, lactitol, and erythritol) into your carb limit calculations. On the other hand, each gram of sorbitol, isomalt, maltitol, or glycerin counts as about 0.5 gram of carbs. Further, fiber are all listed under carbs but our body can't process them; they do not have an energy value for the human body. They are generally listed under "Dietary Fiber" on food labels. Soluble dietary fiber plays a key role in the regulation of appetite by achieving stabilized insulin levels. Further, the key to healthy low-carb dieting is to learn about macronutrients and how they affect your body. Thus, you should consider calculating your net carbs rather than total carbs. If you are a beginner, watch out for hidden carbs.

Consider energy density.

In fact, energy density is the number of calories per gram of food. As for a keto diet, it is advisable to base your diet plan around medium energy density foods and eat higher energy density foods in small amounts. On the other hand, lower energy density foods have fewer calories per gram of food. They include clear soups and stews as well as vegetables and simple garden salads that are naturally high in water.

Eat real food.

This means that on a ketogenic diet you'll need to eat whole, unprocessed food that is rich in nutrients. It is extremely important to avoid chemical additives and junk food. Focusing on whole, organic and grass-fed foods will make your life easier and your body healthier.

3 Proven Benefits of a Ketogenic Diet

1) A keto diet leads to weight loss. When you avoid carbohydrates, your body starts burning stored fat; it will automatically cause decreased appetite. On the other hand, you will experience higher energy levels.

3) **Mental clarity and better concentration.** On a keto diet, our brain uses ketones as the main fuel; consequently, it reduces the levels of toxins. It will significantly improve your cognitive functions, mental focus, concentration, and mental performance.

2) **Health benefits.** A keto diet restricts carbohydrates; they can be found in unhealthy sugary foods, refined grains such as bread, pasta and white rice. On the other hand, it promotes foods that are loaded with high-quality protein (it is essential for building muscle), good fat, and healthy veggies. Many studies have proven that low-carb diets can significantly improve health. They measured the main outcomes such as LDL cholesterol, HDL cholesterol, blood sugar levels, triglycerides, and weight loss.

Fatty fish such (for example, tuna and salmon) is well known for its ability to lower triglycerides; consequently, it can reduce the risk of stroke. Unsaturated fat-packed foods such as seeds, nuts and unrefined vegetable oils can help your body to lower triglycerides, too. In addition, cutting out carbs can reduce insulin levels and regulate blood sugar. Not only can keto diets improve your physical performance and boost weight loss, but they also treat some serious conditions. Keto diets have proven beneficial in treating several brain disorders such as epilepsy in children. Moreover, ketogenic diets are incredibly effective in treating metabolic syndrome.

A Few Hacks You Might Benefit From

Stay hydrated – According to the United States National Library of Medicine, an adult person should drink between 2.7 to 3.7 liters of water per day. Be careful of liquid calories on a ketogenic diet. Avoid alcohol and sweetened drinks; you can satisfy your thirst with sparkling water (with added fresh lemon juice), full-fat yogurt, or ice tea. Eat fresh vegetables that are naturally high in water content. As many keto-ers, I experienced dry mouth and bad breath, too; they are common symptoms of ketosis. How I get rid of ketosis breath? The trick is to brush regularly, chew sugar-free gum, and drink more water.

Fat coffee – This is my little secret to burning fat faster. A cup of coffee with a tablespoon of butter gives me a prolonged energy hit until lunchtime. I love its creaminess and distinctly aftertaste and I am impressed by its results. It may sound crazy, but try it once and you will fall in love with "fat black".

Keep it simple – The key to a successful ketogenic diet is making simple tweaks to your lifestyle. Make a simple ketogenic meal plan to get yourself into a routine; stick to easy recipes such as salads and soups. Go for simple snacks, too. Declutter and simplify your kitchen, and choose quick meals to cook at home. Let go of control, relax and go outside. Getting fresh air and spending time with family or pets will help make you more likely to stick to your diet.

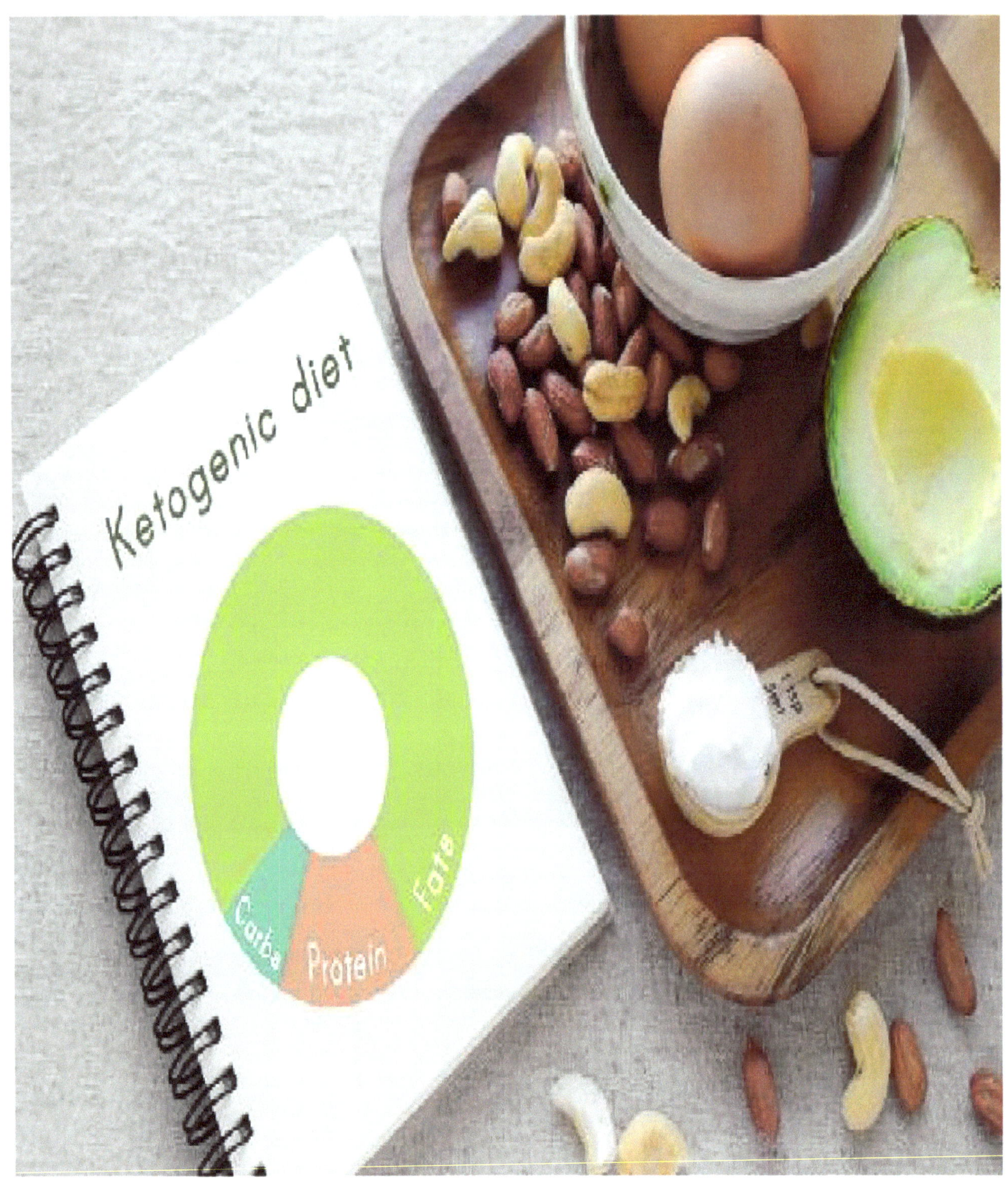

21-Day Meal Plan

I created an easy-to-follow meal plan for you to kick-start your keto journey right. This is a sample menu for three weeks on a ketogenic diet plan.

DAY 1

Breakfast – 1 tablespoon of peanut butter; 1 slice of keto bread **Lunch** – Easy Turkey Curry; 1 handful of iceberg lettuce **Dinner** – Smoked Haddock Fish Burgers; 1 medium tomato DAY 2

Breakfast – 1 hard-boiled egg; 1 slice of bacon; 1 shake with 1/2 cup of coconut milk and protein powder **Lunch** – Classic Beef Stroganoff; 1 serving of cauliflower rice **Dinner** – Alaskan Cod with Mustard Cream Sauce; 1 medium tomato DAY 3

Breakfast – Paprika Omelet with Goat Cheese; 5-6 almonds **Lunch** – Chinese Ground Beef Skillet; 1 cup raw baby spinach with apple cider vinegar **Dinner** – Special Chicken Salad; 1 keto dinner roll DAY 4

Breakfast – Omelet with veggies; 1 slice of bacon **Lunch** – Pork Cutlets in Chili Tangy Sauce; 1 serving of coleslaw **Dinner** – Lemon Garlic Grilled Chicken Wings; 1 medium tomato DAY 5

Breakfast – Dilly Boiled Eggs with Avocado; a dollop of sour cream; 1-2 pickles **Lunch** – Beef Shredded Beef with Herbs; 1 handful of mixed green salad with a few drizzles of a freshly squeezed lemon juice **Dinner** – Two-Cheese Zucchini Gratin; 1 teaspoon of mustard DAY 6

Breakfast – Greek-Style Frittata with Herbs; 1 keto roll **Lunch** – Holiday Pork Belly with Vegetables; 1 serving of cauliflower rice **Dinner** – Ranch and Blue Cheese Dip; Greek-style salad (tomato, cucumber, bell peppers, feta cheese) DAY 7

Breakfast – Mangalorean Egg Curry **Lunch** – Italian Zuppa di Pomodoro; 1 large tomato; 1 cup of fried mushrooms with 1 tablespoon of butter **Dinner** – Ranch Chicken Wings; Cheese and Artichoke Dip DAY 8

Breakfast – Scrambled eggs; 1 tomato; 1/2 cup of Greek-style yogurt **Lunch** – Cheeseburger Skillet with Bacon and Mushrooms; 1 serving of cauliflower rice **Dinner** – Swedish Herring Salad DAY 9

Breakfast – Egg, Bacon and Kale Muffins; 1/2 cup unsweetened almond milk **Lunch** – Hearty Fisherman's Stew; 1 serving of cabbage salad **Dinner** – Two-Cheese and Kale Bake DAY 10

Breakfast – Cauliflower, Cheese and Egg Fat Bombs **Lunch** – Grandma's Zucchini and Spinach Chowder; 1/2 chicken breast; 1 scallion **Dinner** – Italian

Cheese Crisps; a dollop of sour cream; 2 tablespoons tomato paste DAY 11

Breakfast – 1 tablespoon of peanut butter; 1 slice of keto bread **Lunch** – Country-Style Pork Stew; 1 serving of cabbage salad **Dinner** – Cauliflower, Ham and Cheese Bake DAY 12

Breakfast – The Best Zucchini Fritters Ever; 1/2 cup of full-fat Greek yogurt **Lunch** – Filipino Nilaga Soup; 1 serving of low-carb grilled vegetables **Dinner** – Peanut Butter Cubes DAY 13

Breakfast – Crêpes with Peanut Butter and Coconut **Lunch** – Creamy Broccoli and Bacon Soup; 1 medium cucumber; 1 roasted chicken drumstick **Dinner** – Mexican-Style Pork Tacos DAY 14

Breakfast – Vanilla Mug Cake **Lunch** – Cheesy Zucchini Casserole; 1 handful of baby spinach with 1 teaspoon of mustard and 1 teaspoon of olive oil **Dinner** – Turkey Crust Pizza with Bacon DAY 15

Breakfast – Easiest Brownies Ever **Lunch** – Salmon Curry with a Twist; 1 serving of roasted keto veggies **Dinner** – Stuffed Spaghetti Squash Bowls DAY 16

Breakfast – Deviled Eggs with Mustard and Chives; 1/2 cup of Greek-style yogurt **Lunch** – Ranch Chicken Breasts with Cheese **Dinner** – Spicy Baked Eggplant with Herbs and Cheese; Almond Butter and Chocolate Cookies DAY 17

Breakfast – 2 hard-boiled eggs; 2 slices of Cheddar cheese **Lunch** – Pork Tenderloin with Southern Cabbage; 1 slice of keto bread **Dinner** – Italian-Style Spicy Meatballs; 1 cucumber DAY 18

Breakfast – Lettuce Wraps with Ham and Cheese **Lunch** – Stuffed Peppers with Cauliflower and Cheese; 1/2 grilled chicken breast **Dinner** – Smoked Haddock Fish Burgers DAY 19

Breakfast – Double Cheese and Sausage Balls **Lunch** – Indian-Style Fried Pork; 1 serving of steamed broccoli; 1 cucumber **Dinner** – 1 grilled pork sausage; 1 teaspoon Dijon mustard; Chinese-Style Cauliflower Rice DAY 20

Breakfast – Cheesy Brussels Sprouts; 1 medium tomato with 2-3 Kalamata olives **Lunch** – Spinach with Paprika and Cheese; 1 dollop of sour cream **Dinner** – Rich Double-Cheese Meatloaf DAY 21

Breakfast – Mini Stuffed Peppers; 1 serving of blue cheese **Lunch** – Holiday Pork Belly with Vegetables; 1 serving of cabbage salad **Dinner** – 1 steamed chicken breast; 1 serving of roasted asparagus; Peanut Butter and Chocolate Treat If you get hungry between meals, there are healthy, keto snacks that can fill you up. They include one or two hard-boiled eggs, baby carrots with tablespoon or two of a keto dipping sauce, full-fat yogurt with tablespoon or two of fresh berries, a handful of nuts, and a few cheese sticks.

All about Our Recipe Collection

My goal with this book is to support and inspire people who decide to make a positive change in their lives. For that reason, this book features 75 recipes, from simple recipes for new keto-ers to festive recipes that everyone will love, so that you never run out of ideas.

All of these recipes are made with common ingredients that deliver great flavor and stunning aromas. They are approved by my husband and my guests who often come over for dinner. They are designed to guide you every step of the way in order to prepare the best keto foods ever. Each recipe includes the nutritional information and has up to 6 grams of net carbs. This is the best way to track your macronutrients and customize your diet to fit your unique needs. Besides being a great source for keto recipes, the book is chock-full of cooking secrets, crafty tricks, and handy hacks. Are you ready to go keto? Go ahead! Remember, if I can do it, you can too!

VEGETABLES & SIDE DISHES

1. Cauliflower, Ham and Cheese Bake

(Ready in about 40 minutes | Servings 4)

This creamy casserole tastes so divine! Cauliflower combines beautifully with ham, cheese, Greek-yogurt and Mediterranean herbs.

Per serving: 188 Calories; 11.3g Fat; 5.7g Carbs; 1.1g Fiber; 14.9g Protein; 2.9g Sugars *Ingredients*

1/2 teaspoon butter, melted 1 (1/2-pound) head cauliflower, broken into florets 1/2 cup Swiss cheese, shredded 1/2 cup Mexican blend cheese, room temperature 1/2 cup Greek-style yogurt 1 cup cooked ham, chopped 1 roasted chili pepper, chopped 1/2 teaspoon porcini powder 1 teaspoon garlic powder 1 teaspoon shallot powder 1/2 teaspoon cayenne pepper 1/4 teaspoon dried sage 1/2 teaspoon dried oregano Sea salt and ground black pepper, to taste *Directions*

Start by preheating your oven to 340 degrees F. Then, coat the bottom and sides of a casserole dish with 1/2 teaspoon of melted butter.

Empty the cauliflower into a pot and cover it with water. Let it cook for 6 minutes until it is nice and tender (mashable). Mash the prepared cauliflower with a potato ricer press or potato masher.

Now, stir in the cheese; stir until the cheese has melted. Add Greek-style yogurt, chopped ham, roasted pepper, and spices.

Place the mixture in the prepared casserole dish; bake in the preheated oven for 20 minutes. Let it sit for about 10 minutes before cutting. Serve and enjoy!

2. Creamy Broccoli and Bacon Soup

(Ready in about 20 minutes | Servings 4)

This creamy soup will help you keep your diet on track. It can be refrigerated up to 3 days.

Per serving: 95 Calories; 7.6g Fat; 4.1g Carbs; 1g Fiber; 3g Protein; 1.7g Sugars
Ingredients

2 slices bacon, chopped 2 tablespoons scallions, chopped 1 carrot, chopped 1 celery, chopped Salt and ground black pepper, to taste 1 teaspoon garlic, finely chopped 1/2 teaspoon dried rosemary 1 sprig thyme, stripped and chopped 1/2 head green cabbage, shredded 1/2 head broccoli, broken into small florets 3 cups water 1 cup chicken stock 1/2 cup full-fat yogurt ***Directions***

Heat a stockpot over medium heat; now, sear the bacon until crisp. Reserve the bacon and 1 tablespoon of fat.

Then, cook scallions, carrots, and celery in 1 tablespoon of reserved fat. Add salt, pepper, and garlic; cook an additional 1 minute or until fragrant.

Now, stir in rosemary, thyme, cabbage, and broccoli. Pour in water and stock, bringing to a rapid boil; reduce heat and let it simmer for 10 minutes more.

Add yogurt and cook an additional 5 minutes, stirring occasionally. Use an immersion blender, to puree your soup until smooth.

Taste and adjust the seasonings. Garnish with the cooked bacon just before serving.

3. Spinach with Paprika and Cheese

(Ready in about 10 minutes | Servings 4)

Make a popular side dish in 10 minutes and amaze your guests! Other common additions to this recipe include Parmesan cheese, nutmeg and herbs.

Per serving: 166 Calories; 15.1g Fat; 5g Carbs; 1.7g Fiber; 4.4g Protein; 2.1g Sugars ***Ingredients***

1 tablespoon butter, room temperature 1 clove garlic, minced 10 ounces spinach 1/2 teaspoon garlic salt 1/4 teaspoon ground black pepper, or more to taste 1/2 teaspoon cayenne pepper 3 ounces cream cheese 1/2 cup double cream
Directions

Melt the butter in a saucepan that is preheated over medium heat. Once hot. Cook garlic for 30 seconds.

Now, add the spinach; cover the pan for 2 minutes to let the spinach wilt. Season with salt, black pepper, and cayenne pepper Stir in cheese and cream; stir until the cheese melts. Serve immediately.

4. Cheesy Zucchini Casserole

(Ready in about 50 minutes | Servings 4)

This is a great way to use up the bounty of zucchini during the summer season. You're going to love this easy cheese casserole!

Per serving: 155 Calories; 12.9g Fat; 3.5g Carbs; 0.8g Fiber; 7.6g Protein; 0.2g Sugars ***Ingredients***

Nonstick cooking spray 2 cups zucchini, thinly sliced 2 tablespoons leeks, sliced 1/2 teaspoon salt Freshly ground black pepper, to taste 1/2 teaspoon dried basil 1/2 teaspoon dried oregano 1/2 cup Cheddar cheese, grated 1/4 cup heavy cream 4 tablespoons Parmesan cheese, freshly grated 1 tablespoon butter, room temperature 1 teaspoon fresh garlic, minced ***Directions***

Start by preheating your oven to 370 degrees F. Lightly grease a casserole dish with a nonstick cooking spray.

Place 1 cup of the zucchini slices in the dish; add 1 tablespoon of leeks; sprinkle with salt, pepper, basil, and oregano. Top with 1/4 cup of Cheddar cheese. Repeat the layers one more time.

In a mixing dish, thoroughly whisk the heavy cream with Parmesan, butter, and garlic. Spread this mixture over the zucchini layer and cheese layers.

Place in the preheated oven and bake for about 40 to 45 minutes until the edges are nicely browned. Sprinkle with chopped chives, if desired. Bon appétit!

5. Stuffed Peppers with Cauliflower and Cheese

(Ready in about 45 minutes | Servings 6)

Above ground vegetables such as bell pepper and cauliflower are generally good keto options while below ground vegetables contain more carbs. These peppers are delicious served hot or cold. Enjoy!

Per serving: 244 Calories; 12.9g Fat; 3.2g Carbs; 1g Fiber; 16.5g Protein; 1.6g Sugars *Ingredients*

2 tablespoons vegetable oil 2 tablespoons yellow onion, chopped 1 teaspoon fresh garlic, crushed 1/2 pound ground pork 1/2 pound ground turkey 1 cup cauliflower rice 1/2 teaspoon sea salt 1/4 teaspoon red pepper flakes, crushed 1/2 teaspoon ground black pepper 1 teaspoon dried parsley flakes 6 medium-sized bell peppers, deveined and cleaned 1/2 cup tomato sauce 1/2 cup Cheddar cheese, shredded *Directions*

Heat the oil in a pan over medium flame. Once hot, sauté the onion and garlic for 2 to 3 minutes.

Add the ground meat and cook for 6 minutes longer or until it is nicely browned. Add cauliflower rice and seasoning. Continue to cook for a further 3 minutes.

Divide the filling between the prepared bell peppers. Cover with a piece of foil. Place the peppers in a baking pan; add tomato sauce.

Bake in the preheated oven at 380 degrees F for 20 minutes. Uncover, top with cheese, and bake for 10 minutes more. Bon appétit!

6. Chinese-Style Cauliflower Rice

(Ready in about 15 minutes | Servings 3)

This Asian-style omelet with cauliflower is full of healthy keto foods. You can add some chilli for an extra kick, if desired.

Per serving: 131 Calories; 8.9g Fat; 6.2g Carbs; 1.8g Fiber; 7.2g Protein; 2.2g Sugars ***Ingredients***

1/2 pound fresh cauliflower 1 tablespoon sesame oil 1/2 cup leeks, chopped 1 garlic, pressed Sea salt and freshly ground black pepper, to taste 1/2 teaspoon Chinese five-spice powder 1 teaspoon oyster sauce 1/2 teaspoon light soy sauce 1 tablespoon Shaoxing wine 3 eggs ***Directions***

Pulse the cauliflower in a food processor until it resembles rice.

Heat the sesame oil in a pan over medium-high heat; sauté the leeks and garlic for 2 to 3 minutes. Add the prepared cauliflower rice to the pan, along with salt, black pepper, and Chinese five-spice powder.

Next, add oyster sauce, soy sauce, and wine. Let it cook, stirring occasionally, until the cauliflower is crisp-tender, about 5 minutes.

Then, add the eggs to the pan; stir until everything is well combined. Serve warm and enjoy!

7. Spicy Baked Eggplant with Herbs and Cheese

(Ready in about 2 hours 45 minutes | Servings 6)

Eggplant is baked between layers of Italian cheese, kale, and garlic-tomato pasta sauce, making this Italian-inspired meal oh-so-delicious! You can add a few sprinkles of other Italian spices such as parsley and sage, if desired. You can also garnish your dish with fresh herbs for an extra flavor and even better presentation.

Per serving: 230 Calories; 18.5g Fat; 6.7g Carbs; 2.4g Fiber; 10.6g Protein; 3.3g Sugars ***Ingredients***

1 (3/4-pound) eggplant, cut into 1/2-inch slices 1 tablespoon olive oil 1 tablespoon butter, melted 8 ounces kale leaves, torn into pieces 14 ounces garlic-and-tomato pasta sauce, without sugar 1/3 cup cream cheese 1 cup Asiago cheese, shredded 1/2 cup Gorgonzola cheese, grated 2 tablespoons ketchup, without sugar 1 teaspoon Peperoncino (hot pepper) 1 teaspoon Basilico (basil) 1 teaspoon oregano 1/2 teaspoon Rosmarino (rosemary) ***Directions***

Place the eggplant slices in a colander and sprinkle them with salt. Allow it to sit for 2 hours. Wipe the eggplant slices with paper towels.

Brush the eggplant slices with olive oil; cook in a cast-iron grill pan until nicely browned on both sides, about 5 minutes.

Melt the butter in a pan over medium flame. Now, cook the kale leaves until wilted. In a mixing bowl, combine the three types of cheese.

Transfer the grilled eggplant slices to a lightly greased baking dish. Top with the kale. Then, add a layer of 1/2 of cheese blend.

Pour the tomato sauce over the cheese layer. Top with the remaining cheese mixture. Sprinkle with seasoning.

Bake in the preheated oven at 350 degrees F until cheese is bubbling and golden brown, about 35 minutes. Bon appétit!

8. The Best Zucchini Fritters Ever

(Ready in about 40 minutes | Servings 6)

These fritters are quick and easy to whip up for dinner. Serve with a dollop of sour cream, if desired. You can serve them as a side, too.

Per serving: 111 Calories; 8.9g Fat; 3.2g Carbs; 1g Fiber; 5.8g Protein; 0.5g Sugars ***Ingredients***

1 pound zucchini, grated and drained 1 egg 1 teaspoon fresh Italian parsley 1/2 cup almond meal 1/2 cup goat cheese, crumbled Sea salt and ground black pepper, to taste 1/2 teaspoon red pepper flakes, crushed 2 tablespoons olive oil ***Directions***

Mix all ingredients, except for the olive oil, in a large bowl. Let it sit in your refrigerator for 30 minutes.

Heat the oil into a non-stick frying pan over medium heat; scoop the heaped tablespoons of the zucchini mixture into the hot oil.

Cook for 3 to 4 minutes; then, gently flip the fritters over and cook on the other side. Cook in a couple of batches.

Transfer to a paper towel to soak up any excess grease. Serve and enjoy!

9. Stuffed Spaghetti Squash Bowls

(Ready in about 1 hour | Servings 4)

All the flavors of your favorite pasta are packed into these edible bowls, but they are keto-friendly and guilt-free! These bowls look really fancy, they are suitable for any occasion.

Per serving: 219 Calories; 17.5g Fat; 6.9g Carbs; 0.9g Fiber; 9g Protein; 4.1g Sugars ***Ingredients***

1/2 pound spaghetti squash, halved, scoop out seeds 1 teaspoon olive oil 1/2 cup Mozzarella cheese, shredded 1/2 cup cream cheese 1/2 cup full-fat Greek yogurt 2 eggs 1 garlic clove, minced 1/2 teaspoon cumin 1/2 teaspoon basil 1/2 teaspoon mint Sea salt and ground black pepper, to taste ***Directions***

Place the squash halves in a baking pan; drizzle the insides of each squash half with olive oil.

Bake in the preheated oven at 370 degrees F for 45 to 50 minutes or until the interiors are easily pierced through with a fork Now, scrape out the spaghetti squash "noodles" from the skin in a mixing bowl. Add the remaining ingredients and mix to combine well.

Carefully fill each of the squash half with the cheese mixture. Bake at 350 degrees F for 5 to 10 minutes, until the cheese is bubbling and golden brown. Bon appétit!

10. Tangy Classic Chicken Drumettes

(Ready in about 40 minutes | Servings 4)

A ketogenic dinner doesn't have to be complicated. Simple ingredients – chicken, lemon, garlic. Minimal work—maximum pay-off!

Per serving: 209 Calories; 12.2g Fat; 0.4g Carbs; 0.1g Fiber; 23.2g Protein; 0.1g Sugars ***Ingredients***

1 pound chicken drumettes 1 tablespoon olive oil 2 tablespoons butter, melted 1 garlic cloves, sliced Fresh juice of 1/2 lemon 2 tablespoons white wine Salt and ground black pepper, to taste 1 tablespoon fresh scallions, chopped ***Directions***

Start by preheating your oven to 440 degrees F. Place the chicken in a parchment-lined baking pan. Drizzle with olive oil and melted butter.

Add the garlic, lemon, wine, salt, and black pepper.

Bake in the preheated oven for about 35 minutes. Serve garnished with fresh scallions. Enjoy!

11. Easy Turkey Curry

(Ready in about 1 hour | Servings 4)

Ginger powder is loaded with health benefits, while a curry paste makes your food tastes so good. You can also add herbed salt, paprika, chives, and other spice blends.

Per serving: 295 Calories; 19.5g Fat; 2.9g Carbs; 0g Fiber; 25.5g Protein; 3.1g Sugars ***Ingredients***

3 teaspoons sesame oil 1 pound turkey wings, boneless and chopped 2 cloves garlic, finely chopped 1 small-sized red chili pepper, minced 1/2 teaspoon turmeric powder 1/2 teaspoon ginger powder 1 teaspoon red curry paste 1 cup unsweetened coconut milk, preferably homemade 1/2 cup water 1/2 cup turkey consommé Kosher salt and ground black pepper, to taste ***Directions***

Heat sesame oil in a sauté pan. Add the turkey and cook until it is light brown about 7 minutes.

Add garlic, chili pepper, turmeric powder, ginger powder, and curry paste and cook for 3 minutes longer.

Add the milk, water, and consommé. Season with salt and black pepper. Cook for 45 minutes over medium heat. Bon appétit!

12. Ranch Chicken Breasts with Cheese

Per serving: 295 Calories; 19.5g Fat; 2.9g Carbs; 0g Fiber; 25.5g Protein; 3.1g Sugars ***Ingredients***

2 chicken breasts 2 tablespoons butter, melted 1 teaspoon salt 1/2 teaspoon garlic powder 1/2 teaspoon cayenne pepper 1/2 teaspoon black peppercorns, crushed 1/2 tablespoon ranch seasoning mix 4 ounces Ricotta cheese, room temperature 1/2 cup Monterey-Jack cheese, grated 4 slices bacon, chopped 1/4 cup scallions, chopped ***Directions***

Start by preheating your oven to 370 degrees F.

Drizzle the chicken with melted butter. Rub the chicken with salt, garlic powder, cayenne pepper, black pepper, and ranch seasoning mix.

Heat a cast iron skillet over medium heat. Cook the chicken for 3 to 5 minutes per side. Transfer the chicken to a lightly greased baking dish.

Add cheese and bacon. Bake about 12 minutes. Top with scallions just before serving. Bon appétit!

13. Cheesy Chicken Drumsticks

(Ready in about 20 minutes | Servings 2)

Chicken, spices, lots of cheese… what's not to love about these low-carb, creamy drumsticks? Peanut oil has a high smoke point; you can use unrefined sunflower oil and avocado oil, too.

Per serving: 589 Calories; 46g Fat; 5.8g Carbs; 1g Fiber; 37.5g Protein; 3.8g Sugars ***Ingredients***

1 tablespoon peanut oil 2 chicken drumsticks 1/2 cup vegetable broth 1/2 cup cream cheese 2 cups baby spinach Sea salt and ground black pepper, to taste 1/2 teaspoon parsley flakes 1/2 teaspoon shallot powder 1/2 teaspoon garlic powder 1/2 cup Asiago cheese, grated ***Directions***

Heat the oil in a pan over medium-high heat. Then cook the chicken for 7 minutes, turning occasionally; reserve.

Pour in broth; add cream cheese and spinach; cook until spinach has wilted. Add the chicken back to the pan.

Add seasonings and Asiago cheese; cook until everything is thoroughly heated, an additional 4 minutes. Serve immediately and enjoy!

14. Special Chicken Salad

(Ready in about 1 hour 20 minutes | Servings 3)

You can add boiled eggs to the salad just like grandma used to make. You can also use leftover chicken from a roast chicken.

Per serving: 400 Calories; 35.1g Fat; 5.6g Carbs; 2.9g Fiber; 16.1g Protein; 2.2g Sugars ***Ingredients***

1 chicken breast, skinless 1/4 mayonnaise 1/4 cup sour cream 2 tablespoons Cottage cheese, room temperature Salt and black pepper, to taste 1/4 cup sunflower seeds, hulled and roasted 1/2 avocado, peeled and cubed 1/2 teaspoon fresh garlic, minced 2 tablespoons scallions, chopped ***Directions***

Bring a pot of well-salted water to a rolling boil.

Add the chicken to the boiling water; now, turn off the heat, cover, and let the chicken stand in the hot water for 15 minutes.

Then, drain the water; chop the chicken into bite-sized pieces. Add the remaining ingredients and mix well.

Place in the refrigerator for at least one hour. Serve well chilled. Enjoy!

15. Turkey Crust Pizza with Bacon

(Ready in about 35 minutes | Servings 4)

This delicious low-carb pizza is much better than takeout. Other topping ideas include pepperoni, spinach, onion, and marinara sauce. Enjoy!

Per serving: 360 Calories; 22.7g Fat; 5.9g Carbs; 0.7g Fiber; 32.6g Protein; 2.7g Sugars *Ingredients*

1/2 pound ground turkey 1/2 cup Parmesan cheese, freshly grated 1/2 cup Mozzarella cheese, grated Salt and ground black pepper, to taste 1 bell pepper, sliced 2 slices Canadian bacon, chopped 1 tomato, chopped 1 teaspoon oregano 1/2 teaspoon basil *Directions*

In mixing bowl, thoroughly combine the ground turkey, cheese, salt, and black pepper.

Then, press the cheese-chicken mixture into a parchment-lined baking pan. Bake in the preheated oven, at 390 degrees F for 22 minutes.

Add bell pepper, bacon, tomato, oregano, and basil. Bake an additional 10 minutes and serve warm. Bon appétit!

16. Old-Fashioned Chicken Soup

(Ready in about 55 minutes | Servings 6)

This no-noodle chicken soup is hearty and delicious when it's cold outside. It will be a huge hit during the winter season!

Per serving: 265 Calories; 23.8g Fat; 4.3g Carbs; 1.7g Fiber; 9.3g Protein; 2.3g Sugars ***Ingredients***

1 rotisserie chicken, shredded 6 cups water 2 tablespoons butter 2 celery stalks, chopped 1/2 onion, chopped 1 bay leaf Sea salt and ground black pepper, to taste 1 tablespoon fresh cilantro, chopped 2 cups green cabbage, sliced into strips
Directions

Cook the bones and carcass from a leftover chicken with water over medium-high heat for 15 minutes. Then, reduce to a simmer and cook an additional 15 minutes. Reserve the chicken along with the broth.

Let it cool enough to handle, shred the meat into bite-size pieces.

Melt the butter in a large stockpot over medium heat. Sauté the celery and onion until tender and fragrant.

Add bay leaf, salt, pepper, and broth, and let it simmer for 10 minutes.

Add the reserved chicken, cilantro, and cabbage. Simmer for an additional 10 to 11 minutes, until the cabbage is tender. Bon appétit!

17. Crispy Chicken Filets in Tomato Sauce

(Ready in about 15 minutes | Servings 3)

The key to this recipe is to crush the pork rinds in a Ziploc bag by hand, since we need a panko-like texture. A simple tomato sauce goes along very well with chicken.

Per serving: 359 Calories; 23.6g Fat; 5.8g Carbs; 1.2g Fiber; 30.4g Protein; 3.1g Sugars ***Ingredients***

2 tablespoons double cream 1 egg 2 ounces pork rinds, crushed 2 ounces Romano cheese, grated Sea salt and ground black pepper, to taste 1 teaspoon cayenne pepper 1 teaspoon dried parsley 1 garlic clove, halved 1/2 pound chicken fillets 2 tablespoons olive oil 1 large-sized Roma tomato, pureed ***Directions***

In a mixing bowl, whisk the cream and egg.

In another bowl, mix the crushed pork rinds, Romano cheese, salt, black pepper, cayenne pepper, and dried parsley.

Rub the garlic halves all over the chicken. Dip the chicken fillets into the egg mixture; then, coat the chicken with breading on all sides.

Heat the olive oil in a pan over medium-high heat; add ghee. Once hot, cook chicken fillets until no longer pink, 2 to 4 minutes on each side.

Transfer the prepared chicken fillets to a baking pan that is lightly greased with a nonstick cooking spray. Cover with the pureed tomato. Bake for 2 to 3 minutes until everything is thoroughly warmed. Bon appétit!

18. Lemon Garlic Grilled Chicken Wings

(Ready in about 25 minutes + marinating time | Servings 4)

For a quick dinner on busy weeknights, place some chicken wings and marinade in a Ziploc bag; freeze them and Voila! On an actual day, thaw them and place on the preheated grill.

Per serving: 131 Calories; 7.8g Fat; 1.8g Carbs; 0.2g Fiber; 13.4g Protein; 0.4g Sugars *Ingredients*

8 chicken wings 2 tablespoons ghee, melted The Marinade: 2 garlic cloves, minced 1/4 cup leeks, chopped 2 tablespoons lemon juice Salt and ground black pepper, to taste 1/2 teaspoon paprika 1 teaspoon dried rosemary *Directions*

Thoroughly combine all ingredients for the marinade in a ceramic bowl. Add the chicken wings to the bowl.

Cover and allow it to marinate for 1 hour.

Then, preheat your grill to medium-high heat. Drizzle melted ghee over the chicken wings. Grill the chicken wings for 20 minutes, turning them periodically.

Taste, adjust the seasonings, and serve warm. Enjoy!

PORK

19. Mexican-Style Pork Tacos

(Ready in about 20 minutes | Servings 4)

You could serve this pork mixture on a bed of zucchini noodles. Other popular fixings include shredded cheese, guacamole, Tabasco sauce, mustard, tomato, and bell peppers.

Per serving: 330 Calories; 26.3g Fat; 4.9g Carbs; 1.3g Fiber; 17.9g Protein; 2.4g Sugars ***Ingredients***

6 ounces ground pork 4 ounces ground turkey Sea salt and ground black pepper, to taste 1 tablespoon lard 4 tablespoons roasted tomatillo salsa 12 lettuce leaves 4 tablespoons fresh cilantro, chopped 4 tablespoons sour cream ***Directions***

In a mixing bowl, thoroughly combine the ground pork, turkey, salt, and black pepper.

Melt the lard in a skillet over medium-high heat. Once hot, cook the meat mixture for 5 to 6 minutes, crumbling with a fork.

Add the roasted tomatillo salsa and stir to combine well.

To assemble the tacos, divide the salsa-meat mixture between lettuce leaves. Top with cilantro and sour cream. Make wraps and serve immediately.

20. Pork Cutlets in Chili Tangy Sauce

(Ready in about 15 minutes | Servings 4)

These pork cutlets are perfectly seasoned and cooked with lots of herbs. Finally, they are served with a spicy sherry sauce.

Per serving: 288 Calories; 17.3g Fat; 1.1g Carbs; 0g Fiber; 29.9g Protein; 0.1g Sugars ***Ingredients***

1 pound pork cutlets Sea salt and ground black pepper, to taste 1/2 teaspoon thyme 1/2 teaspoon rosemary 1 teaspoon basil 1 tablespoon lard, room temperature The Sauce: 2 tablespoons sherry 1/4 cup sour cream 1/4 cup beef bone broth 1 teaspoon mustard 1/2 teaspoon turmeric powder 1/2 teaspoon chili powder ***Directions***

Season the pork cutlets with salt, pepper, thyme, rosemary, and basil.

Melt the lard in a pan over medium-high heat; now, sear pork cutlets for 3 minutes; turn them over and cook for 3 minutes on the other side. Reserve.

Deglaze your pan with sherry; now, add the remaining ingredients and cook on medium-low heat until the sauce has thickened slightly.

Add the reserved pork and let it simmer for a couple of minutes or until everything is heated through. Spoon the sauce over pork cutlets and serve.

21. Holiday Pork Belly with Vegetables

(Ready in about 20 minutes | Servings 4)

Are you thinking about an oven roasted crispy pork? Look no further! This pork belly is tender with amazing crispy skin.

Per serving: 607 Calories; 60g Fat; 4.4g Carbs; 0.7g Fiber; 11.4g Protein; 2.1g Sugars ***Ingredients***

1 pound skinless pork belly Himalayan salt and freshly ground black pepper, to taste 1 teaspoon dried parsley 1 teaspoon dried basil 1/2 teaspoon dried oregano 2 cloves garlic, pressed 1/2 cup shallots, sliced 1 red bell pepper, seeded and sliced 1 green bell pepper, seeded and sliced ***Directions***

Poke holes all over the pork with a fork. Rub the seasonings all over the pork belly. Place the pork in a lightly greased baking pan.

Top with garlic, shallots, and peppers. Transfer the pork belly to the preheated oven.

Bake at 390 degrees F for about 18 minutes. Serve warm.

22. Cheeseburger Skillet with Bacon and Mushrooms

(Ready in about 20 minutes | Servings 4)

Are you craving cheeseburgers but you do not have the time to cook them? No worries, this amazing dish comes together in one skillet in less than 20 minutes.

Per serving: 463 Calories; 60g Fat; 4.7g Carbs; 0.8g Fiber; 36.2g Protein; 3g Sugars ***Ingredients***

2 slices Canadian bacon, chopped 1/2 cup shallots, sliced 1 garlic clove, minced 1 pound ground pork Sea salt and ground black pepper, to taste 1/3 cup vegetable broth 1/4 cup white wine 6 ounces Cremini mushrooms, sliced 1/2 cup cream cheese ***Directions***

Heat a cast-iron skillet over medium heat. Cook the bacon for 2 to 3 minutes; reserve the bacon and 1 tablespoon of fat. Then, sauté the shallots and garlic in 1 tablespoon of bacon fat until tender and fragrant.

Add the ground pork, salt, and black pepper to the skillet. Cook for 4 to 5 minutes or until ground meat is nicely browned.

Add broth, wine, and mushrooms. Cover and cook for 8 to 9 minutes over medium flame.

Turn off the heat. Add cream cheese and stir to combine. Serve topped with the reserved bacon. Enjoy!

23. Country-Style Pork Stew

(Ready in about 40 minutes | Servings 4)

Per serving: 351 Calories; 22.7g Fat; 2.7g Carbs; 0.5g Fiber; 32.3g Protein; 1.5g Sugars ***Ingredients***

2 tablespoons lard, room temperature 1/4 cup leeks, chopped 2 garlic cloves, minced 1 (1-inch) piece ginger root, peeled and chopped 1 bell pepper, seeded and chopped 1 pound pork stew meat, cubed 1/2 cup tomato paste 2 cups chicken broth Sea salt and ground black pepper, to taste 1 teaspoon paprika 1 bay leaf 1/4 cup Creme fraiche ***Directions***

Melt the lard in a sauté pan that is preheated over medium heat. Then, cook the leeks, garlic, and ginger until aromatic, about 3 minutes.

Add bell pepper and cook for a further 2 minutes, stirring periodically. Add the pork and cook an additional 3 minutes or until no longer pink.

Stir in the tomato paste, broth, salt, pepper, paprika, and bay leaf. Cover and let it simmer over low-medium heat approximately 30 minutes.

Stir in Creme fraiche; turn off the heat and stir until everything is well combined. Ladle into serving bowls and serve immediately.

24. Cheesy and Buttery Pork Chops

(Ready in about 20 minutes | Servings 2)

If you are short on time, these pork chops with cheese, spices and butter are faster than ordering takeout. You can use any full-fat, firm cheese of your choice.

Per serving: 494 Calories; 39.8g Fat; 5.3g Carbs; 1.1g Fiber; 28.6g Protein; 2.7g Sugars ***Ingredients***

1/2 stick butter, room temperature 1/2 cup white onion, chopped 4 ounces button mushrooms, sliced 1/3 pound pork loin chops 1 teaspoon dried parsley flakes Salt and ground black pepper, to taste 1/2 cup Swiss cheese, shredded ***Directions***

Melt 1/4 of the butter stick in a skillet over medium heat. Then, sauté the onions and mushrooms until the onions are translucent and the mushrooms are tender and fragrant, about 5 minutes. Reserve.

Then, melt the remaining 1/4 of the butter stick and cook pork until slightly browned on all sides, about 10 minutes.

Add the onion mixture, parsley, salt, and pepper. Lastly, top with cheese; cover and let it cook on medium-low heat until cheese has melted.

Serve immediately and enjoy!

25. Filipino Nilaga Soup

(Ready in about 45 minutes | Servings 4)

You can use a slow cooker to cook this soup; cook on high for 4 hours or until the meat is fork-tender. You can also add beef chuck roast or ribs and cook it all together.

Per serving: 203 Calories; 8.4g Fat; 3.7g Carbs; 1.1g Fiber; 27.1g Protein; 1.7g Sugars ***Ingredients***

1 teaspoon butter 1 pound pork ribs, boneless and cut into small pieces 1 shallot, chopped 2 garlic cloves, minced 1 (1/2-inch) piece fresh ginger, chopped 1 cup water 2 cups chicken stock 1 tablespoon patis (fish sauce) 1 cup fresh tomatoes, pureed 1 cup cauliflower "rice"

Sea salt and ground black pepper, to taste ***Directions***

Melt the butter in a pot over medium-high heat. Then, cook the pork ribs on all sides for 5 to 6 minutes.

Add the shallot, garlic and ginger; cook an additional 3 minutes. Add the remaining ingredients.

Let it cook, covered, for 30 to 35 minutes. Ladle into individual bowls and serve.

26. Pork Tenderloin with Southern Cabbage

(Ready in about 25 minutes | Servings 2)

You can marinate pork for a foolproof tenderloin if desired. Professional cooks add a bit of lemon juice to the cabbage while cooking.

Per serving: 254 Calories; 10.8g Fat; 5.7g Carbs; 1.6g Fiber; 31.8g Protein; 3.3g Sugars *Ingredients*

The Pork tenderloin: 1/2 pound pork tenderloin Celtic sea salt and freshly cracked black pepper, to taste 1/2 teaspoon granulated garlic 1/4 teaspoon ginger powder 1/2 teaspoon dried sage 1 tablespoon lard, room temperature The Cabbage: 4 ounces cabbage, sliced into strips 1/3 cup vegetable broth 2 tablespoons sherry wine 1/2 teaspoon mustard seeds Celtic sea salt, to taste 1/2 teaspoon black peppercorns *Directions*

Season the pork with salt, black pepper, granulated garlic, ginger powder, and sage.

Melt the lard in a pan over moderate heat. Sear the pork for 7 to 8 minutes, turning periodically.

In a pan that is preheated over medium heat, bring the cabbage, broth, sherry, and mustard seeds to a boil over high heat.

Season with salt and black peppercorns; cook, stirring periodically, until the cabbage is tender, about 12 minutes; do not overcook.

Serve the pork with sautéed cabbage on the side. Bon appétit!

27. Indian-Style Fried Pork

(Ready in about 15 minutes | Servings 4)

Pork shoulder is the perfect cut for this recipe; it has a great meat to fat ratio. Serve with mashed cauliflower and you will have a perfect ketogenic, family meal.

Per serving: 478 Calories; 34.7g Fat; 2.2g Carbs; 0g Fiber; 36.4g Protein; 0.3g Sugars *Ingredients*

1 teaspoon shallot powder 1 teaspoon porcini powder 1 teaspoon garlic powder 1/2 teaspoon cumin 1/4 teaspoon turmeric powder 1 cinnamon stick 2 dried Kashmiri red chillies, roasted Sea salt and ground black pepper, to taste 1 pound pork shoulder 1/2 cup ground pork rinds 1/2 cup Parmesan cheese, grated 2 eggs 2 tablespoons tallow *Directions*

Blend the spices together with the cinnamon and chillies until you have a smooth paste. Rub this paste all over the pork shoulder.

In a bowl, combine the pork rinds with parmesan cheese. In a separate bowl, whisk the eggs.

Slice the pork into small pieces; dip the pork in the egg and then, cover it with the pork rind mixture.

Melt the tallow in a skillet over medium-high heat. Cook the pork for 2 to 3 minutes per side. Bon appétit!

www.ingramcontent.com/pod-product-compliance
Lightning Source LLC
Chambersburg PA
CBHW042001110726
48006CB00004B/952